Disclaimer

The information in this eBook reflects the opinions of the author and is not intended to replace medical or psychological advice, or any other professional advice. This EBook is not intended to diagnose or treat any psychological or medical conditions or disorders. If you are in need psychological or medical treatment, consult with a certified and licensed professional before determining whether the information in this book should be used.

No More Pimples – Solution Revealed

Table of Contents

No More Pimples – Solution Revealed

Top 10 Acne Fighting Foods

You are what you eat, isn't it? But, it's crazy to believe that eating pizzas, chocolates and other junk food items gives you acne! No doubt, these foods contribute to acne flare-ups but there are many other factors like hormones, genes, skin type, environmental impact and your skincare routine that could give you the zits. Interestingly, as certain foods contribute to flare ups, there are some food pyramid items that help fight acne.

Here are 10 acne fighting foods that can give you clearer skin:

Omega 3 fatty acids – Salmon, Flax seed, Walnuts: Omega 3 fatty acids are considered wondrous for the skin. These help in keeping skin inflammation at bay and keep acne under control. Two servings of fatty fish such as salmon, mackerel or sardines a week or a tablespoon of flaxseed or walnuts in your salads and smoothies can up your Omega power.

Foods rich in selenium – Brazil nuts, Onion, Garlic, Whole grains: Brazil nuts are the perfect source of selenium which is a very powerful antioxidant. It helps in controlling acne and preserves the skin's elasticity. It also reduces inflammatory damage to the skin. One Brazil nut a day is power packed for a days' supply of selenium. Follow selenium intake with Vitamin A and E to pack in more acne fighting punch.

Foods rich in Vitamin C – Melons, Oranges, and Tomatoes: Add enough Vitamin C to your diet to boost your immune system and strengthen your cell walls. Though these foods will not directly impact acne they will definitely help in protecting your skin from acne scarring. The bioflavonoids coming from this vitamin C source are natural anti inflammatories and enhance Vitamin C's healing power.

Foods rich in Vitamin E – Almonds, Leafy greens, Eggs: Vitamin E is an antioxidant that helps the skin to heal from acne damage and scarring. However, if you are on a low fat diet it might not be easy to source the requisite amount of Vitamin E. Try minimally processed oils such as canola oil to get the requisite dose of Vitamin E. An ounce of almonds, spinach drizzled with a tablespoon of olive oil or an egg daily can give you the required Vitamin E.

Foods high in water content – Watermelons, Cucumbers, Parsley: If you are suffering from acne you will always be advised to up your water intake. Foods that have a high water content such as cucumbers, watermelons, parsley, romaine lettuce, cabbage help in keeping your system free from toxins. Eat your water and get clear skin!

Foods rich in beta carotene – Carrots, Bell peppers, Cantaloupes, Sweet potatoes: Foods such as carrots, cantaloupes, sweet potatoes and other yellow, orange and red fruits and vegetables are very high in beta carotene. Beta carotene converts to Vitamin A in the body and enhances the benefits of selenium to the skin. Aim to introduce at least ½ a cup of yellow or red fruits and veggies to your daily diet.

Foods high in magnesium: Foods high in magnesium such as bananas, artichokes, buckwheat, oats, brown rice, figs are great acne fighters since magnesium helps to balance the acne inducing hormones.

Green tea: Polyphenols and flavonols contained in green tea are very powerful antioxidants that help in reducing oxidation damage caused by free radicals. Green tea consumption inhibits bacterial colonization, contains hormonal activity and sooths inflammation.

Watch the sodium: Iodized salt and other strong sources of iodine for some reason cause acne to flare up. Watch out for your sodium intake in processed or prepared food. Skip to sea salt since it has a lower iodine content.

Black out the white stuff: When you want to scale off acne then scale off the white stuff. White bread, white rice, white refined flour, French fries, mashed potatoes and other refined stuff made from sugar are seriously off limits. Blood sugar causes insulin to spike which in turn causes acne flare ups.

I understand the strife and pain we all go through with zits and pimples. We just don't like one popping-up! Integrate these 10 foods in your diet to stay healthy, vibrant and skin healthy- heal yourself with the right food.

7 Secrets that Cured My Acne without Chemicals

7 secrets to cure acne without chemicals, natural acne cures

For those wondering, no that is not me. It's a stock photo :)

While I do focus on grain-free, food related topics, I wanted to share these tips that have make a huge difference in my chronic acne. After all, Empowered Sustenance covers things that sustain and empower us. And I think these natural cures for acne does both!

All I ever wanted for Christmas was clear skin…

Acne and I: inseparable since 7th grade. It requires pages to explain the myriad of treatments, lotions, potions and prescriptions under my belt. Basically, I've tried every prescription besides Acutane and birth control pills (and I will never touch those). Everything from drugstore cleansers to $90 serums have graced my medicine cabinet. I've even invested in at-home peel chemical peels, a Clarisonic, and laser treatments.

Natural acne treatments that work!

I've discussed how starting the SCD/GAPS diet made changes in my skin. Unfortunately, my improved facial acne situation was still considered "severe." I've been experimenting with this specific combination of natural acne treatments and I think I've discovered what is going to permanently treat my acne.

I went cold turkey on all my skin care products–albeit "natural" products–and have been using the following, homemade regimen for about a month. While my acne is not completely gone, I know with a bit more time this routine will cure my acne.

1. Oil Cleansing in the Evening

I was apprehensive about smothering my face with oil, since my face has always been veritable oil slick one hour after I wash it. So it took a big dose of courage to throw out my face wash and tried this method for oil cleansing. I love it! It removes all traces of makeup and leaves my skin soft.

Most importantly, my face's oil production is normalizing. This is because–in conjunction with the facial oil I'll talk about–it does not need to overcompensate with oil production like it did when I cleansed with soap.

2. Honey Cleansing in the Morning

In the mornings, I wash my face with honey. With slightly dampened fingers, I massage about 1/2 teaspoon of raw honey over my dry face and then rinse. The antibacterial properties of honey work to inhibit breakouts. Additionally, it removes excess oil but leaves skin moisturized. You can read more details on my post The Honey Cleansing Method.

3. Apple Cider Vinegar Toner for Acne

Mornings and evenings, I spray my face with a mixture of 2/3 alcohol free which hazel and 1/3 raw apple cider vinegar. The apple cider contains gentle exfoliating acids to calm acne and it balances the skin's pH. It also allows my homemade facial oil to absorb quickly and evenly.

4. Homemade Acne Facial Oil

I use a twist on Crunchy Betty's formula for facial oil. I fill a 1 oz. jar with jojoba oil then add a few drops of carrot seed oil. The jojoba oil dissolves excess sebum without over-drying the skin, and the carrot seed oil is extremely reparative and healing for the skin.

I just moisten my face with the toner, warm a few drops of this oil mixture between my fingertips and massage lightly onto my face. As a bonus, it feels like a quick aromatherapy treatment.

natural acne cure, natural acne treatment5. Honey, Cinnamon and Nutmeg Spot Treatment

If you ever visit my house without giving me prior warning, you might just see me walking around with dots of gooey cinnamon on my zits. This is my normal routine ever since discovering that this mask makes a super effective spot treatment.

I mix raw honey with enough cinnamon to form a paste, add some freshly grated nutmeg, and store it in a small container in my bathroom. I'll leave this spot treatment on for a couple of hours. If you want to use it as a full face mask, leave it on for only 10-15 minutes.

6. Baking Soda Exfoliant

Once a week, I mix up a paste of baking soda and water and apply it to my face, chest, and back. I leave it on for a few minutes before my bath or shower. It provides gentle chemical exfoliation to even skin tone, dry up breakouts, and eliminate blackheads. As a bonus, this effective treatment is simple and economical!

UPDATE: I no longer recommend this exfoliation because it can be too harsh for the skin due to the strong alkalinity of baking soda. You must be extremely careful in selecting exfoliants for the face and chest because the skin is so delicate. Sugar scrubs, salt scrubs, apricot-hull scrubs and the rest are all much to harsh and can lead to premature aging. Even enzyme peels and acid peels are usually too harsh for the skin and disrupt the acid mantle.

7. Acupuncture for Acne and Hormone Balance

7 secrets to cure acne without chemicalsBefore starting the GAPS diet, my health was so poor that I rarely got periods. GAPS brought my cycle back, but also delivered intense PMS. I'm talking nausea, headaches, and doubling over in pain from cramps. Desperate for a solution, I gave acupuncture a try. After two months of weekly treatment, my periods are getting better and better.

So how does this relate to acne? During that time of the month, my skin usually erupts into landscape of deep, painful cystic acne. Since starting the acupuncture treatment, I've noticed a marked improvement in PMS breakouts. I am going to continue regular acupuncture to see if my periods will continue to improve, and I think it will continue to reduce my hormonal acne.

UPDATE: Imbalanced hormones were absolutely the main cause behind my acne and cystic acne. After many, many hours of research and self-experimentation, I have learned how to balance my hormones naturally through dietary, lifestyle and supplemental changes. My cystic acne and PMS is now a thing of the past! I share all the resources and instructions to end PMS in my new ebook Quit PMS: End Your Menstrual Misery.

8. Bonus! Enessa Clove Acne Control for Cystic Acne

Yes, so the title says 7 things. But I had to update this post with a #8 because I couldn't believe I had forgotten this! I rely onEnessa Clove Acne Control to reduce cystic acne (the deep and painful hormonal acne). This is the only topical treatment I've found that drastically reduces the inflammation and redness of cysts overnight. I always have an extra bottle around because I cannot bear to run out of this magic potion.

Enessa Clove Acne Control is a secret blend of clove oil and other essential oils in a base of jojoba oil. Do not go out and by a bottle of clove essential oil and think it will do the same thing. As a matter of fact, putting straight clove oil on your skin will burn and damage the skin, because it is so strong. The Enessa product may be a bit pricey, but it works... so it is a worthwhile investment for me.

Why go the natural route for acne?

These homemade acne cures may seem crazy, but it is not as crazy as dousing one's face in toxic, stripping, chemical-based products. Normalizing the skin's oil production, using gentle spot treatments and exfoliation and (for the ladies) balancing period hormones through acupuncture means a safe and effective solution to acne.

Are you passionate about effective skin care without toxic ingredients? Then use the buttons below to share these tips!

Back To School Tips On How To Prevent Acne And Break-Outs

Tweet

3

back-to-school2-300x190It is that time of the year again. School is starting and for many it means dealing with one of the most difficult skin condition: acne. Typically, acne clears up nicely during the summer when people are outdoors and under less stress, but a month after school begins pimples and blackheads start to pop up again. Although acne is a problem that most often affects young people, many people in their 40s and 50s still experience it. Oily skin, hormones, genetics, improper skin care and stress can all contribute to the problem, making outbreaks worse. Although you may not be able to completely eliminate acne, proper skin care can help to prevent acne outbreaks.

Here are 5 tips on how to prevent breakouts:

1, Don't touch your face! You probably don't even realize that you're doing it. Siting at your desk and resting your face on your hand can cause breakouts. All the dirt, oil and bacteria that build up on your hands during the day will end up on your face and clog your pores. Make a conscious effort to keep your hands off your face and stop picking at your skin.

2, Change your pillowcase more often! During the night your skin will detoxify itself so all the toxins, oils and hair products can end up on your pillowcase. By changing your sheets and pillowcase once or twice a week will help keep your skin clear.

3, Wash your face twice every day to prevent pimples, blackheads and whiteheads. Use a facial cleanser for acne prone skin and wash your face gently to avoid irritating your skin. Include your neck, back, shoulders and any other areas affected by acne. Don't wash too often, as excessive rubbing can over dry your skin and make your acne worse.

4, Don't cram for exams: Reading papers, tons of projects and homework can wrack havoc on your skin.Study a little every day to avoid stressing out before your test. Stress is one of the biggest contributors for acne. Make sure to take some time for yourself every day to relax.

5, Eat nutritious foods that will keep you and your skin healthy. Eat a variety of whole grains, fruits and vegetables, but use sugar, fried foods, dairy and highly-processed foods in moderation. Although foods are not the main cause of acne, but there are certain triggers such as dairy and salt that is proven to create lot's of inflammation in the skin. Drink plenty of water. At least 8 large glasses of water every day will keep your skin hydrated and will prevent dryness from the exfoliating acne products.

Top 12 Very Simple Tips to avoid Pimples

1 year agoAashima SinghPeople & Lifestyle12 Comments

To look attractive it is not just about good clothes but an attractive skin is also desirable. Each one of us wants a fresh and clear skin with no sign of wrinkles or blemishes over it. And what about pimples? Oh we so loathe them. Pimples are in fact one of the most stressful things to spot in morning. They are red, they are ugly and they can also be infectious. For a lot of people pimples are a complete nightmare. Imagine this- A romantic date with your boyfriend and a night before there is this little red monster sitting on your forehead or you have got an important board meeting at office but an evil pimple on your nose can draw more attention than your PowerPoint presentation. Nightmares aren't these? The moment we spot a pimple on our face we start thinking of all the possible ways to get rid of it as soon as possible. But getting rid of pimples isn't that an easy task as we may think or maybe it is! Here are 12 simplest of tips which you can follow and these will definitely help in keeping your skin pimple free.

12. Keep your face clean

keep your face clean

Cleansing shall be one of the most important steps of your skin care routine. Even if you are not having an acne problem washing the face twice a day helps in removing dirt, oil and dead skin cells from the surface of your skin. Less oil and dirt also means less acne. While washing your face never apply soap and always use a mild face cleanser. Also wash the face only with warm or cold water as using hot water can cause pimples.

11. Watch your hair often

wash your hair

To avoid having pimples it is not just necessary to keep your face oil free but your hair shall also not be oily. Leaving overnight oil on your hair can cause pimples as the hair touching your face will make your skin oily. Wash your hair regularly and don't let them fall on your face. Also go easy on products like hair gels, fragrances and deodorants as they can clog up the skin pores leading to pimples.

10. Keep your hands away from your face

keep your hands away

Siting an unpleasant pimple makes us want to pop it immediately to get rid of it. But touching and popping pimples can only accentuate the problem. Don't let your hands touch your face very often. It can spread bacteria, cause infections or further more pimples which you certainly don't want.

9. Eat healthy

eat healthy

Mothers always tell us that no amount of cosmetic products can benefit our skin as much as eating a healthy diet comprising of fresh fruits and vegetables can. This is in fact true. Eating oily and greasy food like chocolates or junk food doesn't do much good to our skin while eating grains, fruits and vegetables helps us in keeping it healthy and pimple free.

8. Apply ice

apply ice

Ice soothes the skin, particularly the affected area which can help your skin to become pimple-free. Applying ice on the skin will remove the oil and dirt trapped inside and reduces the redness and swelling. To get rid of an eruption, put an ice cube in a cloth and gently press it against the affected skin. Or one can also make it a routine to apply crushed ice or ice cubes to the skin in order to avoid pimples.

7. Apply honey

apply honey

Honey masks are quite a common acne treatment. Applying honey on the face works both as a preventive method and as a treatment for pimples. It is a natural antiseptic that soothes and heals the skin. The antioxidants present in honey can help in reducing the inflammation over the skin and making it pimple free. Apply some honey on your face for 15-30 minutes and then wash it off. Not only will it work against your acne problem but it also makes the skin smooth and supple.

6. Use lemons

use lemon

Like honey, lemons are also believed to be a quite effective natural treatment for getting rid of pimples. Lemons can help avoiding pimples in more than one way. Lemon juice reduces the oil, kills bacteria, reduces redness and also removes the pimple scars. To use it over your pimples squeeze some fresh lime juice over a cotton swab or a cotton ball and apply it over your face. It can give quick results.

5. Use baking soda

use baking soda

Another wonder product which you already have in your kitchen and it can help you fight against pimples is baking soda. A mixture of baking soda and lemon juice can be applied on the skin to make it pimple free. Baking soda is an amphoteric compound which means it can work both as an acid and as a base. It helps in neutralizing the skin's pH, imbalance in which is often a cause behind acne. It also dries the skin removing any extra oil and mixing some baking soda with water works wonderfully in cleansing and exfoliating our skin.

4. Apply toothpaste

apply toothpaste

While treating pimples you don't always need to go and buy some specialized cosmetic product but your humble toothpaste can also be of a lot of use. Now while using toothpaste as a pimple treatment always choose a white toothpaste and not the gel or red, blue or green stripes ones. Also don't use the teeth whitening toothpaste to apply over the skin. Wash your face with warm water and a cleanser and pat dry. Now take a pea size amount of toothpaste and apply it only over the affected area. Keep it for a couple of hours or overnight and then wash it. Your pimples must be either gone or much less visible.

3. Use Aloe Vera

use aloe vera

Aloe Vera is a cactus like plant with anti-bacterial, anti-fungal, anti-septic, astringent and a lot more useful medicinal properties. It can be used in a lot of ways- as a moisturizer, a face mask, shaving oil or it can also be included in your diet. Aloe Vera can work wonders for treating and preventing acne as it removes excess oil and dirt from the skin. It stimulates the cell growth, and helps the damaged skin for healing faster.

2. Use dermatological products or treatments

use dermatological products or treatments

If all else fails then this can be your backup plan. There is a huge variety of anti-acne products- face washes, creams, face packs etc., available in the market these days. Search a little, find a product that will best suit your skin type and give it a try. If still your pimples are unlikely to go away then don't hesitate from going to a dermatologist.

1. Take a chill pill!

take a chill pill

If you didn't know it already then let me break it to you. Stress causes PIMPLES!! Not that I'm excited about it or something but it actually does. When our body produces the stress hormone, it leads to causing pimples in two ways. 1: The hair follicle lining thickens due to the hormone causing whiteheads and blackheads and if bacteria gets trapped inside of it, a pimple is formed. 2: Our body directs blood and oxygen to more vital areas leaving skin dehydrated and prone to clogged pores and breakouts. Hence in order to avoid pimples one also needs to reduce their stress levels. You may try yoga or meditation to stay stress-free and pimple-free.

Pimples are a very common skin issue that affects people of different ages. Excessive oil secretion from the oil glands present in the skin is certainly one of the primary reasons of pimples. When the skin pores are clogged due to dead skin cells or dirt this secreted oil is accumulated under the skin and the painful pimple emerges due to bacterial infection on these oil glands.

There are some characteristic differences between acne and pimples. While pimples are considered as of lesser frequency; acne is referred as a chronic skin condition and can be of different types. Hormones and other physical reasons can be a cause of pimples, rarely, but most of the times, they are caused due to not cleaning the skin properly and also due to use of skin care and makeup products that does not suit the skin type. It has also been found that in case of acne, heredity might play an indirect role.

Some people have an idea that pimples occur over the face only; but, it is not always right. Pimples can affect any area of the skin like shoulders, back, hands as well as legs. Pimples may not be a serious disease but can portray a negative impression about the person, hampering his/her self-esteem and image.

Environmental pollution, exposure to sun, use of cosmetics, excessive stress, junk foods and inadequate water intake are some of the common reasons that directly or indirectly triggers break outs of pimples.However, do not panic!!!We have some good kitchen secrets and tips that can help you immensely to cure pimples without making a hole in your pocket. Here we go.

Home remedies for pimple marks & scars

Natural home remedies to get rid of pimples

Products that are readily available in your kitchen can work amazingly and are more promising than the pre-packed store bought masks for fighting pimples.

Aloe Vera gel to stop pimples

Aloe Vera gel can work magically on pimples. It is a skin soothing and purifying agent that can be effective to treat pimples quickly. Prepare some fresh Aloe Vera pulp from an Aloe Vera leaf and apply it directly onto the pimples and leave on. Do not wash until it dries up completely.

Baking soda

How to use baking soda to reduce pimples? Baking soda is packed with anti-fungal and antiseptic properties and it can control pimples effectively. Mix 1 tsp of baking soda with few drops of water to make a thick paste. Apply this paste directly onto the pimples. Wash off with normal water after 5 minutes.

Home remedies for acne marks

How to use toothpaste to remove pimples

Toothpaste can also be effective home remedy to get rid of pimples. Apply a small drop of toothpaste onto the pimple before going to the bed and wash it off with cold water in the morning. Observe the results. This is the best method to get rid of pimples instantly. Do no use gel tooth paste; use any white tooth paste.

Tea tree oil to treat pimples

Tea tree oil is a strong antibacterial agent, it can fight pimples efficiently. Mix 2-3 drops of tea tree oil with 4-5 drops of carrier oil (primrose oil is a good option for pimples) and apply the mixture directly onto the pimples. Leave on for 15-20 minutes. Remove the oil with a damp cotton ball.

Get rid of pimples with garlic paste

Wondering how to get rid of pimples quickly? Try out garlic. Garlic is packed with natural antioxidants and is an effective anti-bacterial agent. Using garlic to reduce pimples can be very effective. Take a few slices of garlic and make a smooth paste. Apply this paste to the pimple and leave on for 10 minutes. Wash off with plenty of water.

Home remedy with Fenugreek seeds

A powder of fenugreek seeds can also be used for curing pimples effectively. Mix fenugreek powder with sufficient water to make a paste and apply the paste onto the pimples. This is the best way to get rid of pimples and pimple marks.

Best acne & pimple soaps

Sandalwood to treat acne & pimple

Sandalwood can help you immensely to get rid of pimples. Use a sandalwood stick for making the paste. Use rose water instead of water while rubbing the stick on the sand stone to make a runny paste. Apply this paste onto the pimples before hitting the bed. In the morning wash it off with cold water.

Quick remedy for pimples with mint

Mint leaves have anti-bacterial properties and they give an effective cooling effect on the skin which can be very helpful to reduce the inflammation caused due to pimples. Take some fresh mint leaves, wash them clean with normal water and make a fine paste. Apply this paste onto the pimples and leave on. Wash off after 20 -30 minutes.

Get rid of pimples fast with neem & basil leaves

Both neem and basil leaves have excellent antibacterial and skin soothing properties. Make a paste of neem and basil leaves and apply it directly onto the pimples. You can also prepare a neem and basil rinse by boiling 10-15 neem and 8-10 basil leaves in water for 15 minutes and then extracting the concoction. Use this concoction to wash your face as many times as you can during a day; and you will get pimple free completely clear skin.

Heal pimples with honey & turmeric

Both honey and turmeric has anti-bacterial and skin soothing properties. A paste made from these two ingredients can be effective to treat pimples. Make a smooth paste of fresh turmeric root and add 5-6 drops of honey to it. Mix well and apply this paste onto the pimples. Let it set for 30 minutes or more and then wash off with plain water.

Acne & pimple control creams

Papaya pack to reduce pimple marks

Here is one best natural home remedy for both pimples and pimple marks. Papaya is rich in anti-oxidants and enzymes, which are believed to work on the bacteria causing the pimple. So, using a freshly prepared paste of papaya onto the pimple can be an effective way to reduce the pimple over time. Papaya can also be effective to reduce the pimple marks.

Cucumber

Cucumber is soothing for the skin and being packed with enzymes it can be effective to kill the bacteria infecting the clogged pores. Make a fine paste of cucumber and apply it onto your skin. Leave on for 30 minutes and then wash off with plain water.

Reduce pimples with steaming

Another effective home treatment to remove pimples is steaming. If you have pimples, steam your face so that the pores open up and enable the skin to breathe. The bacteria, dirt and oils trapped in the skin pores can be removed by lightly scrubbing your face after steaming. Consider it to be the best way to reduce pimples.

Tips for preventing pimple break outs

It is always said that prevention is better than cure and in fact you can prevent pimples easily, because they are not usually caused due to hormonal reasons. All you need to do is to take a bit extra care for your skin.

Take up a regular skin care regime

Resort to a 2 times daily cleansing-toning-moisturizing regime. For cleansing, use some mild cleanser or simply some homemade cleanser. For toning you can use the neem-basil rinse as mentioned above or only rose water. For moisturizing, use any herbal product that absorbs quickly into your skin without leaving any residue or stickiness.Exfoliate your skin properly with a homemade scrub like coffee-honey scrub at least twice a week to ensure that there is no dead cell build up on the skin that can clog the pores.

Multani mitti face packs for acne & pimples

Stay away from chemicals

Today, whatever products you buy from stores including cleansing lotions, face wash, moisturizers, night creams, sunscreens, make up items, almost every product you use on a daily basis has chemicals in it which may pose many skin related issues in the long run. Try to avoid using many chemical products by replacing face washes, toners and cleansers with homemade products. If you are getting frequent pimple break outs, it might be due to the makeup products you use. Opt for high quality mineral based makeup products or light makeup to ensure that the chemicals of these makeups are not working as the cause of the break outs.

Do not touch face with dirty hands

Most of the times it is our own hands, riding on which the bacteria reaches our face and causes the pimples. So, don't touch your face with uncleaned hands. It can cause the infection at the first place and can even exaggerate the condition.

22 Home Remedies for Acne & Pesky Pimples

acneYour skin is your friend. You like your skin. Your skin likes you. It protects you from the elements and literally keeps you together. You in turn do your best to protect it from any kind of damage. Then, one day, acne rears its ugly head, and you suddenly hate your skin. What do you do then? Turn to harsh chemicals, and expensive scrubs? That's a fine way to thank a friend who's been there for you since day one. Your epidermis isn't at fault here-it can't help that your hormones are causing all that extra sebum to clog up your pores, or the fact that bacteria is running rampant. If your skin could talk it would say something along the lines of "patience, grasshopper. Treat me right and I shall repay you in kind."

That's just a guess, anyways. The point is, natural acne remedies are a good way to get rid of it, or at least hold it at bay. They make you step back and really figure out what's going on with your skin, and how to work with it. Chances are, your skin will repay you in kind for not simply ravaging it with strange chemicals-and your wallet will probably thank you too.

1. Apply some apple cider vinegar

Apple cider vinegar is a powerhouse when it comes to acting as an acne remedy. Why? It kills off the bacteria that may be causing all the trouble in the first place. It also becomes alkaline, and balances the pH of your skin, which in turn makes it harder for bacteria to thrive. To top it off it's an astringent, like lemon juice, and will help dry up excess oil. Keeping that in mind, don't overdo and dry out your skin too much. This could cause the sebaceous glands overproduce to compensate, therefore triggering an outbreak.

You will need…

-Pure unfiltered apple cider vinegar

-Fresh water

Directions

Wash your face with water and pat dry. Using a ratio of 1 part vinegar to 3 parts water, dip a cotton ball into vinegar and apply it directly to the blemish. Leave on for at least 10 minutes, or overnight. Reapply several times a day, washing face thoroughly after each time. Make sure to use a moisturizer afterwards as well if you feel like your skin is getting dry.

Apply Some Apple Cider Vinegar

2. Make a cinnamon and honey mask

Honey is sticky, and cinnamon is spicy, and it seems like they're both things you'd want to avoid getting near your skin. Surprisingly, while it may sound strange, honey and cinnamon make a (literally) killer combo when it comes to acne. Cinnamon has antimicrobial properties, so it can help stop bacteria from getting out of hand. If it does, the honey is a natural anti-biotic, ready and waiting to wipe the little buggers out.

You will need…

-2 tablespoons of honey

-1 teaspoon of cinnamon

- paper towels

Directions

Rinse your face with water and pat dry. Mix 2 tablespoons of honey and 1 teaspoon of cinnamon together until they are thoroughly blended and have formed a sort of paste. Apply the mask to your face (or spot treat) and leave on for 10-15 minutes. Rinse off completely, and pat your face dry. This is a sticky mixture, so make sure you have some paper towels at on hand.

3. The land of milk and honey (or yogurt)

While there is quite a bit of hub bub around dairy products causing acne, applied topically it seems that milk can improve your outbreaks and skin tone. The reason it is suggested that milk would cause acne is because of the extra hormones in it-but unless it's ingested, this doesn't really do much. For the most part, it just soothes the irritated skin, and helps tone down the redness. Cleopatra swore on the milk baths she took, and well, she was Cleopatra. You could also use yogurt. The acids in it are antibacterial while the fat provides moisture, making it quite nourishing for skin.

You will need...

- 1 tablespoon plain low-fat or full-fat yogurt or milk, anything but skim

- 1 tablespoon of natural, raw, honey

Directions

Let yogurt or milk come to room temperature (or close to) so you don't get a chilly shock when you put it on your skin. Mix 1 tablespoon of milk or yogurt thoroughly with 1 tablespoon of honey. You can apply the mixture with a cotton pad, but scooping it up and patting it on works just fine as well. Let each layer dry before adding a new one, until the mask is the thickness you want. Let it sit for 10-15 minutes. Wash your mask off and use a washcloth to gently scrub in a circular motion, getting rid of loosened dead skin. Once you're finished, moisturize as usual.

Homemade Yogurt & Honey Acne Remedy

4. Whip up some 'whites

Egg whites are an easy and affordable way to help reduce acne and fade scars left by unfortunate blemishes. The reason people have found egg whites to be helpful for their skin is because they're chock full of proteins and vitamins that both combat acne, and help to rebuild your skin cells. They also soak up excess oil, which means excess sebum, (exactly what you were thinking right?) which means less stuff for bacteria to feed on. Hooray! Just make sure to use a good moisturizer afterwards, as they can dry your skin out a bit.

You will need...

-2 to 3 egg whites, separated from yolks

-Bowl

-Washcloth

Directions

Rinse your face with water and pat dry. Separate the whites from the yolks. You can use as many as you like, but normally 2 to 3 is enough. Whisk the whites until they're frothy, and let them sit for a few minutes. Cover your face with the mixture (applying with fingertips is easy) focusing on problem spots. 3 to 4 layers is usually enough, but make sure to wait the first has dried before applying more. Allow the mask to sit and dry for about 20 minutes before rinsing off completely with warm water and a patting dry with a soft washcloth. Apply moisturizer appropriate for your skin type.

5. Papaya for the pimple prone

Papaya is an essential ingredient in a lot of beauty products on the market today, but theres no need to go out of your way to gain its benefits? Plain raw papaya is an all-natural acne remedy that removes dead skin cells and excess lipids from the surface of the skin, leaving it soft and smooth. Lipids are a general term for fats, of which oil is a form of. Papaya also contains an enzyme called papain, which reduces inflammation and helps prevent the pus from forming.

You will need...

-1 fresh papaya

Directions

Rinse your face with water and pat dry. Mash up the flesh of the papaya well, until it is of a consistency that can be easily applied to your skin. Leave it on for 15-20 minutes, and then rinse off completely with warm water. If your skin has a tendency to get dry after you cleanse it, use a moisturizer appropriate for your skin type afterwards.

Papaya

6. Make an orange peel paste

Ah, oranges. They taste rejuvenating and refreshing, and our skin may find them just as appealing as our taste buds do. Acne that is caused by bacteria and extra oil/dead skin cells clogging up pores may improve with the use of an orange peel face mask of sorts, thanks to the vitamin C, citric acid, and it's astringent properties. The vitamin C is particularly helpful because it promotes the growth of new healthy cells, keeping your skin in better condition overall.

You will need…

-2 Orange peels

-Clean, fresh water

Directions

Rinse your face with water and pat dry. Grind/pound up your orange peels (you could use a blender, mortar and pestle, whatever gets the job done) and add a little water to create a paste. Add a little at a time, as too much will make it too thin and runny. Once you have the right consistency, apply it to your face and/or problem areas. Wait for 20-25 minutes. Ideally the mask should be firm, but it can still work if it isn't. Rinse off completely with water, pat your face dry, and apply a good moisturize.

acne

7. Tap into tea tree oil

You'll read about tea tree oil for a lot of home remedies, but will most likely see it mentioned the most when comes to skin care, specifically, acne. But why, when too much oil is clogging the pores and making you break out, would you want to use more oil? Tea tree oil isn't like the oil your skin naturally produces, rather it is more like a solvent that cuts through the extra sebum and dead skin cells, and unblocks the pores. Its antibacterial properties also kill off the acne causing bacteria, and prevent further outbreaks.

Note: Tea tree oil is ok for topical use, but should never be ingested. It should also always be diluted before use.

You will need...

-Tea tree oil (a small bottle will do)

-Clean water

-Q-tips or cotton balls

Directions

Wash your face with water and pat dry. Dilute tea tree oil by mixing 1 part oil to 9 parts water. Dip a Q-tip or cotton swab in mixture, and apply to problem areas. If you decide you want a stronger dilution after a while, you can slowly (slowly!) begin to increase the strength, making sure to use each new mixture for at least a week for making it any stronger. Again, it should never be applied undiluted. You can apply a light moisturizer afterwards if you wish.

Another option, especially if you have sensitive skin, is to dilute it with aloe vera gel instead of water.

Tea Tree Oil

8. Mix strawberries and honey

Honey and strawberries make a home remedy for acne that sounds pretty sweet (pun intended) and it combines two things that are used commonly in pricey, often time's harsh, facial scrubs and cleansers. Strawberries may seem random, but consider the fact that they're high in salicylic acid. Salicylic acid-a primary ingredient in many commercial acne treatments- encourages the epidermis to shed its cells more readily, opening up clogged pores, and neutralizing bacteria. It also shrinks up the pores a little bit, which prevents them from clogging up as much in the future, and encourages new cell growth. Honey also works against bacteria that may be behind your acne, and is an anti-inflammatory.

You will need…

-3 fresh strawberries, washed well

-2 teaspoons of good honey-raw is best

Directions

Wash your face with water and pat dry. Rinse 3 strawberries and mash them up well, taking care that they don't get over-mashed and runny. Add the strawberries to two teaspoons of honey, and thoroughly blend them together. Apply to your face and let the mixture sit for 20 minutes. Rinse off completely with warm water, pat dry, and moisturize if your skin has a tendency to dry out. Use twice a week for at least a month.

9. Utilize a banana peel

Bananas are full of all sorts of goodness-even the part we don't eat. Their peels contain something called lutein, an extremely powerful antioxidant that reduces swelling and inflammation, and encourages healthy cell growth. So…rubbing a banana peel on your face can reduce the redness, obviousness, and discomfort of acne. It's (debatably) a better use than using it to trip your friend.

You will need…

-1 banana peel

Directions

Peel your banana and eat it- it's not cool to waste, and they're good for you. Take the peel, and rub in a circular motion all over your face. When you feel as though you've covered all of your face, let it sit for at least 30 minutes before rinsing it off.

10. Aloe for acne

Aloe vera gel can be used with other things to fight acne, but it's a good thing on its own as well. If it's going to be used on its own, the best is to have a little aloe plant floating around in your house, otherwise a good gel that's sold in stores may work as well-just do some research on which ones have the least amount of additives. Not only is the aloe soothing, it works as an anti-inflammatory, decreasing redness and swelling. It also has antibacterial properties.

You will need...

-Enough aloe vera gel to spot treat or cover your problem areas

Directions

Wash your face with water and pat dry. Using your fingertips or a Q-tip, apply the aloe directly to your problem areas.

11. The wonders of sodium bicarbonate

Sodium bicarbonate, glorious sodium bicarbonate, swoops in and makes itself useful in too many ways to count. In the case of acne remedies, this fabulous substance (also known as baking soda) is useful thanks to its mild antiseptic properties, as well as its uncanny ability to fight off fungus and bacteria and dry up excess oil, all while exfoliating your skin via microdermabrasion and making it soft and beautiful. I know-I get star struck too now whenever I see a box of baking soda.

You will need...

-a box of baking soda

-fresh water

Directions

There are two ways to go about this-making a facial mask, or a straightforward scrub. For a facial mask, mix equal parts baking soda to water to form a thick paste. Massage the paste on in slow circular motions for a 2 minutes. Leave the mask on for around 15-20 minutes, then rinse thoroughly with warm water, pat dry, and moisturize.

For a scrub, mix a half a cup of baking soda with one eighth a cup of water. Apply the paste to your face, massaging it in well. After 5-6 minutes of this, rinse your face thoroughly with warm water, pat dry, and moisturize.

12. Dab some lemon juice on it

Lemon juice can help get rid of breakouts for a number of reasons. It is rich in vitamin C, which is good for all types of skin, and it's a citric acid, so it helps 'exfoliate' the skin as well. Most importantly though, it is an astringent. An astringent will cause a contraction of body tissues, and will therefore dry out the blemish itself. It is also a natural skin whitener, which helps reduce redness. If you misplace a dab you may get a little white spot, but don't panic- it will go away on its own accord. Rinse off any lemon juice before going out in the sun, as it may make you more sensitive to it.

You will need…

-1 tablespoon of freshly squeezed lemon juice (approximately)

-Q-tips or cotton balls (optional)

-Yogurt (optional)

Directions

Rinse face gently with water and pat dry. Dab fingers, a cotton ball, or a Q-tip in lemon juice and apply to pimple. If it stings, try mixing it first with a bit of yogurt.

Dab Some Lemon On It

13. Make it steamy

Steam can help soothe a number of minor maladies, acne being one of them. It helps reduce acne, and its glaring appearance, by opening up the pores and flushing out impurities lurking deep within your skin. You can choose to only steam, or you can use something afterwards. If you use it with something else, you've cleared a sort of path for whatever you're using to really do its job.

You will need...

-1 pot of boiling water

-1 towel

-A large bowl

Directions

Boil a pot of water, pour into a large bowl, and let it cool for a few minutes. After its temperature has lowered slightly, place your face above the bowl, and drape the towel over your head to trap the steam. After 10-15 minutes, remove the towel and pat your face dry. Do this once a day or as needed.

14. The wonders of garlic

Garlic is thought to be a good natural remedy for acne because of its supposed antibacterial properties. You can either ingest it, or apply it topically to help reduce the severity of your breakouts and prevent them in the future. If you can get the juice from the garlic, great, if you can't, mashing it up and putting it in some water is fine. Never, ever, ever, apply garlic to your skin without diluting it first. If you're hesitant about the garlic smell, look at the silver lining-others may be a bit taken aback, but you won't have to worry about Dracula creeping around either.

You will need...

-2-3 cloves of garlic

-water OR aloe vera gel

Directions

Either extract the garlic juice and mix it with 1 teaspoons or so of water, or mash up 2-3 cloves and let sit in water for about 10 minutes. Using a cotton pad, soak up the juice or garlic water and cover problem spots. If you don't have a cotton pad or something similar to apply it with, the mixture can be a bit runny and hard to work with. In this case, substitute aloe vera gel for water. If you choose to ingest garlic, a clove or two a day should be enough. Prepare it however you like.

Garlic Acne Solution

15. Oatmeal boost

Oatmeal can power you up from the inside out-and the outside in. If you soak/cook your oats and use them in mask, they can reduce the inflammation and unsightly redness that accompanies breakouts. Add some honey to your mask and you have a great recipe for a rather tasty sounding acne remedy. Keep in mind that oatmeal on its own will not cure your acne, and should be used as part of a sensible routine acne treatment. However, it may very well reduce the blatant, painful, appearance of the breakouts.

You will need...

-One serving of oatmeal-steel cut seems to work well

-Water

-Two tablespoons raw honey

Directions

Whip up a batch of oatmeal as usual, or by following the directions on the box. When it is finished and still hot, add two tablespoons of honey. Let mixture cool to room temperature. Keep in mind it retains quite a bit of heat, so really make sure it's a comfortable temperature before applying it to your skin-the last thing you need is a burn! Leave it on for 20-30 minutes. When it has set, rinse off with warm water and pat your skin dry.

16. Sugar scrub

Sugar, white or brown, helps get rid of the excess skin cells clogging up your pores by acting as gentle exfoliator. Mix it up with honey, olive oil, or just plain water, and you have a sweet scrub to help rid you of your acne woes. There are plenty of different recipes out there, but we found this one to be particularly delightful (courtesy of cjanecreate.com-thank you for sharing this!)

You will need...

-1 ½ cups of white sugar

-1 ½ cups brown sugar, light or dark

-2-3 tablespoons coarse sea salt

-Roughly 1/2 cup of extra virgin olive oil

-10 tablespoons of pure vanilla extract

-1 whole vanilla bean (totally optional)

Directions

Mix 1 ½ cups of brown sugar and 1 ½ cups of brown sugar, adding in a few tablespoons of coarse sea salt for extra exfoliation, and mix. If you're using the vanilla bean, scrap out the caviar (the inside stuff) and mix it in at this point as well. Put about 2 cups of this sugar/salt/vanilla mixture into a liquid measuring cup and pack it down nice and snug. Pour the extra virgin olive oil over the top, and let it soak through half the mixture, leaving a little layer on top. Mix this up in the measuring cup, and then add it to the rest of the sugar/salt/vanilla mix. Add 4-5 tablespoons of pure vanilla extract and mix it in. Now you can spoon your scrub into whatever containers you wish to store it, making sure to pack it down. If you like, drizzle one tablespoon of vanilla extract on top to ensure that you'll get the delicious scent when you open it up. This will fill 4 half-pint jars.

17. Avocado & honey mask

There are so many rumors surrounding diet and acne, it's hard to know what's right and what's wrong. Amongst these rumors is the claim that avocado (eating it and sometimes applying it topically) will make you breakout, because it's higher in fat. As far as I am concerned, there's no concrete evidence to prove this, and far more people seem to have success using it than not. It's so full of good vitamins and nutrients it seems it can really help tone down the acne. If you have sensitive skin, too, it's quite mild. There are different combinations you can try, as with most home remedies, but this one blends together avocado and honey.

You will need...

-1 avocado

-1 tablespoon of honey

Directions

Rinse your face with water and pat it dry. Scrap out the inside of the avocado and mash it up, then stir in the honey. Continuing mashing/stirring until it turns into a paste. Apply it to your skin and leave it on for 15-20 minutes. When you're done, wash off the mixture with lukewarm water and pat your face dry. Depending on your skin type, apply moisturizer.

Avocado & Honey Mask to Get Rid of Acne

18. Wash your pillowcase

Technically, a pillowcase should be washed at the very least once a week. While most of us don't practice this, when it comes to keeping your skin fresh and healthy, it might help to get a little picky about your pillowcase. If you never wash it, all the stuff that gets rubbed onto it then comes in contact with your face for around 6-8 hours every night, and can exacerbate your acne. Keeping a clean, comfy place to rest your weary head is worth the hassle of stuffing your pillow back into its case-the real reason we avoid washing it-if it could prevent future breakouts.

19. Don't touch your face (more specifically, your breakouts)

This doesn't mean you can rest you chin in your hands or anything-it means don't itch, scratch, pick, peel, pop, or rub at your skin. I distinctly recall the constant discomfort of acne, especially when treating it with irritating topical stuff. Almost subconsciously I would touch my face-probably every 2-3 minutes on average-and pick at my breakouts. Of course, this just made things go from bad to worse. While touching your face with your hands now and then won't cause acne, if you suffer from it, resisting the urge to bug it will help the healing process go smoother and more efficiently.

You will need...

- self control

20. Freshen up with mint

Mint contains menthol, which works as a natural anti-inflammatory and pain killer. It won't cure your acne per say, but it may help the redness fade and ease up some of the discomfort cause by painful swelling.

You will need...

-A decent handful of fresh mint leaves

Directions

Rinse your face with water and pat it dry. Crush up the leaves thoroughly, you can use a blender but a mortar and pestle works quite well if you happen to have one lying around. Rub the juice and crushed leaves on your face and leave for 5-10 minutes before rinsing off thoroughly with cold water.

21. Put a potato on it

Potato is a wonderful vegetable, to be sure, but one of its benefits may not be something you've heard of before. That benefit would be taming acne, as potatoes are full of potassium, sulfur, phosphorus, and chloride-all components that can help reduce bothersome blemishes. They also have antioxidants to nourish your skin and encourage the healthy growth of new skin cells.

You will need...

-1 potato

Directions

Wash your face with water and pat almost dry, leaving it a bit damp. Grate 1 raw potato and rub the pulp and juice onto your face for a few minutes in a circular motion. Let it dry for 15-30 minutes, and then rinse off completely with warm water.

Potato Face Mask

22. Tea Time

There have been some promising studies recently (namely in 2011, 2012, Journal of Investigative Dermatology) in which green tea was shown to have a noticeable impact on acne when used externally. Internally, there is theory it helps as well, but less concrete evidence. To sum up the findings briefly, there is an antioxidant in green tea called epigallocatechin-3-gallate or EGCG. ECGC was shown to reduce sebum production, inflammation, and bacterial growth in acne-prone skin-basically the main causes behind breakouts. It's exciting for the future of acne, or rather, a future without acne. Here's how to use it topically-you can also try drinking a cup or two a day to detoxify.

You will need...

-1/2 cup fresh water

-2 teaspoons loose organic tea leaves OR 1 green tea bag

Directions

Wash your face with water, and pat dry with a soft clean towel. Place your leaves in a clean bowl and pour boiling water over them. Steep for 4-5 minutes before straining the leaves and letting the liquid cool to a comfortable temperature. You can then pour into a spray bottle and spritz your face lightly, soak a cotton pad/soft cloth and apply, or simply use a teabag steeped for 2-3 minutes, patting it onto your face or problem areas. Some people find more success just leaving the refreshing liquid on, while others rinse it off with cool water.

Now what?

Have patience. The desperate urge to find a speedy solution to acne, preferably something that takes minimal effort, is a strong one. In all reality though, and like so many other aspects in life, one really doesn't exist. Having a regular skin care routine and adding a good, natural, acne remedy to it may take extra work, but stay committed, do things right, and give your treatment time to have an effect. Remember, you live in your skin and that's not ever going to change. Taking the effort to really care for it will make all the difference in terms of your comfort, happiness, and confidence.

22 Acne Remedies- to make your skin glow.

Debunking 5 Myths About Acne

Acne is shrouded in misconception, and covered up with conflicting information. Knowing what's true and what's not true can help you figure out how best to treat your skin.

1. Acne is caused by dirt/dirty skin- Acne is not caused by dirt, poor hygiene, not washing your face and so on. Too much scrubbing or cleansing with harsh soaps or chemicals can actually irritate your skin and make the acne worse. If you "over clean" you can end up drying out your skin, which will then try and compensate by making that much more oil. A simple cleansing of the skin to get rid of excess oil and dead skin cells is all that is needed.

2. Greasy food/chocolate makes you breakout-Greasy food and chocolate have been shown to have little to no effect on the development of acne. Diet can still have an impact, as some dairy products or carbs increase blood sugar or have added hormones and trigger acne, but it's not usually the case.

3. Stress causes acne- In theory, stress can affect hormones, and therefore promote acne. It's hard to quantify this though, and when you think about the stress most of us deal with in day to day to life, there wouldnt be an acne free face in sight. An effective acne treatment regime will override a bit of everyday stress anytime.

4. Having acne means you can't use a moisturizer- Look for a good noncomedogenic (meaning less likely to clog pores) moisturizer to use. After treating your acne, be it with banana peels or over the counter creams, a moisturizer can help balance out your skin, ensuring that it doesn't create excess oil to compensate for all that you dried up.

5. Sunlight/tanning clears up acne- In the short term getting a tan, or even slight sunburn, will seemingly clear up your acne. Long term, it's not a solution. It's just hiding the redness, and while it does dry up your skin, it can make it too dry, and do more harm than good.

You may also like our list of 22 Remedies for a Sort Throat

P.S. Take a look at the Everyday Roots Book. It's a Book that we created to help you replace the toxic products and medications in your home with healthier, all-natural alternatives. It contains 215+ effective home remedies and covers everything you will need to protect your family and save money every month.

What Are Pimples?

Pimples are one of the most common skin conditions that you will see in many people especially in teenagers. It is nothing but the inflammation of the skin caused by the attack of bacteria on the sebaceous glands (oil glands). The bacteria infect the skin and this makes the skin to swell up by forming a puss inside. The main reason for the occurrence of pimples is teenagers are due to the excess secretion of sebum by the oil glands during their puberty stage when they undergo a lot of hormonal changes. It normally is seen on the face, neck, back and shoulders. Pimples are not a critical problem at all but it makes you look very miserable and poor in appearance.

Causes Of Pimples

Some of the common causes of pimples are mentioned below:

Pimples are generally caused during puberty and teenage years when there is an increase in the sex hormones and androgen.

Too much consumption of oil and junk foods also causes pimples to easily appear in teenagers.

Hereditary and dirt factors also cause pimples in men and women.

Over use of cosmetic products on the face and inadequate cleansing of these products also causes pimples to appear on the face and neck.

Pressure on the face due to use of helmet straps and so on can also cause pimples.

Accumulation of dead skin cells and overgrowth of bacterial tissues in the body causes pimples.

Symptoms For Pimples

There are no specific symptoms that you will experience to predict that you are going to get pimples on your face or neck or back.

Scaly red skin

Scarring of the skin

Reddish tiny bulbs on your face and neck

Blackheads and whiteheads

Pimples might or might not contain fluid or puss inside

Simple Home Remedies To Treat Pimples

There are many home remedies that you can try out to make a fist of the pimples affecting your skin.

1. Turmeric Powder Paste

Turmeric has antiseptic properties that will fight the bacteria that cause pimples and reduce the production of pimples on the skin.

• Take a tablespoon of turmeric powder and mix it with a few drops of water to make it a thick paste.

• Apply this paste on the affected areas of your face and neck and leave it there for a few minutes.

• Rinse it off with cold water. Repeat this process for five to six days to effectively reduce pimples.

2. Fresh Mint Leaves Juice

Mint leaves are said to have real cooling and antiseptic properties and can work wonders on pimples.

• Take a bunch of fresh mint leaves and grind it to a rough paste form.

• Now squeeze the mint juice out of this paste.

• Apply this mint juice generously all over your face and neck and leave it to rest on the face overnight.

• Wash it off the next day with water and mild soap.

• Repeat this process for four to five days to reduce pimples on face and neck.

3. Lemon Juice

One of the quickest ways to treat pimples is the use of lemon juice. It is rich in Vitamin C and helps to easily dry out pimples.

• Extract 2 tablespoons of lemon juice from two medium sized fresh lemons.

• Dab a generous amount of lemon juice on a cotton ball and apply it to the pimples on your face and neck. Leave it there for 20 minutes and wash it off.

• Repeat this two to three times a day for three to four days to see visible results.

4. Garlic

Garlic is a natural remedy to treat pimples as it has antifungal, antiviral and antiseptic properties. The sulfur in the garlic will help to heal pimples quickly.

• Cut a big clove of garlic into two pieces.

• Now apply the cut end of the garlic on the pimples and leave the juice on the pimples for five minutes.

• Wash this off in lukewarm water and repeat this treatment several times a day to quickly see effective results.

• You can also eat one or two cloves of raw garlic a day to purify your blood and this will help reduce pimples.

5. Toothpaste

Toothpaste that you use to brush your teeth is found to be very effective in treating pimples. You must only use the white toothpaste on your pimples for good results.

• Apply white toothpaste on the affected areas of your face and neck overnight before going to bed.

• Wash your face with water and see if there is some reduction in the size of the pimples.

• You can also do this procedure during day time and make sure that toothpaste remains on the pimples for about one to one and a half hours to see visible results.

6. Steam

Steam is a wonderful treatment for pimples as it will help to open up the pores of the skin and allow the skin to breathe freely. So, the bacteria, dirt and oil trapped in the skin will be easily removed from the skin.

• If you have a steam tub at home, then you need to fill the tub with hot water and allow the steam to come in contact with your face and neck.

• Allow the steam to hit your face for a few minutes.

• Rinse your face now with lukewarm water and pat it dry.

• Repeat this process two times a day for four to five days to reduce pimples and to make skin glow.

7. Ice Pack

Ice is also very effective home remedy for pimples. It removes dirt and oil from skin and also improves blood circulation.

• Wrap ice cubes or crushed ice in a piece of clean cotton cloth and hold it on the pimples on your face and neck or a few minutes.

• Wait for a few minutes and repeat the process three to four times.

• Do this twice a day to see effective results.

Simple Home Remedies To Treat Pimples

8. Cinnamon Powder

• Take one or two teaspoons of freshly ground cinnamon powder and mix it with a tablespoon of honey and lemon juice.

• Make a smooth paste of this mixture and apply on the pimples.

• Leave it there for 20 minutes and wash it off with lukewarm water.

• You can also leave it overnight and wash it off the next day morning to see good results.

9. Orange Peels

• Grind orange peels and mix them with a few drops of water.

• Make it into a paste and apply it on the affected areas of your face.

• Leave it to react with pimples for half an hour and wash it off to see effective results.

10. Honey

Honey is a rich source of natural antibiotics and helps to heal pimples effectively.

• Dip a clean cotton ball in pure honey and apply it generously on the pimples on your face and neck.

• Leave the honey on your pimples for 15 to 20 minutes and wash it off with lukewarm water.

• Repeat the process three times a day to see effective results.

11. Papaya

Papaya is rich in antioxidants and helps in reducing inflammation of the pimples.

• Cut raw papaya into pieces and crush it in a blender.

• Squeeze this paste to extract raw papaya juice and apply this juice over the pimples.

• Leave it for 15 to 20 minutes and then wash it off to see effective results.

12. Cucumber Juice

• Cut cucumber into slices and soak it in drinking water for an hour. All the nutrients and vitamins in the cucumber will get transferred into the water.

• Strain the cucumber water and drink it. Repeat this process two times a day for five days to see visible results.

13. Cucumber Face Mask

• Grind one cucumber into a smooth paste in a blender.

• Add a few drops of honey and lemon juice to cucumber paste and mix it well.

• Apply this mixture on the face as a mask and leave it there for 20 minutes. Rinse it off with warm water. Repeat everyday to see effective results.

14. Apple Cider Vinegar

• Dab a cotton ball in apple cider vinegar and apply it slightly on the affected areas of your face and skin.

• You need to just apply limier amount and you do not need to wash it off.

• Repeat this process once or twice daily to reduce pimples.

15. Tomato Juice

Tomatoes are natural antioxidants and will help in easily removing pimple scars on your skin.

• Cut tomatoes into halves and apply the juicy area of the tomato on the pimples. Hold it for two to three minutes and repeat the same after five minutes.

• Do this twice a day for three to four days to effectively remove pimples.

16. Egg White Face Mask

• Just take the egg white from an egg and apply it generously to the affected areas of your face and skin.

• Leave the paste as long as you can on the pimples or even let it dry on the pimples to see visible results soon.

17. Lavender Oil

• Dip a little bit of lavender oil on a cotton wool and apply it directly on the big pimples on your face and neck.

• Repeat this process often to get rid of pimples soon.

18. Neem Leaves Paste

• Grind neem leaves and then extract its juice. Now add a teaspoon of turmeric powder to this juice and mix well.

• Apply this mixture on the pimples and leave it there for 15 minutes or even overnight.

• Wash it off and repeat every day to get rid of pimples.

Are you worried of reddish and puss filled pimples on your face? Do you find it difficult to move freely in public due to annoying pimples on face? Well, you can get rid of the pimples easily by choosing any of the above effective home remedies.